92 Heartburn Meal and Juice Recipe Solutions:

Prevent Heartburn through All Natural Food Sources

By

Joe Correa CSN

COPYRIGHT

This publication is designed to provide accurate and authoritative information in regard to the subject matter covered. It is sold with the understanding that neither the author nor the publisher is engaged in rendering medical advice. If medical advice or assistance is needed, consult with a doctor. This book is considered a guide and should not be used in any way detrimental to your health. Consult with a physician before starting this nutritional plan to make sure it's right for you.

ACKNOWLEDGEMENTS

This book is dedicated to my friends and family that have had mild or serious illnesses so that you may find a solution and make the necessary changes in your life.

92 Heartburn Meal and Juice Recipe Solutions:

Prevent Heartburn through All Natural Food Sources

By

Joe Correa CSN

CONTENTS

ABOUT THE AUTHOR

After years of Research, I honestly believe in the positive effects that proper nutrition can have over the body and mind. My knowledge and experience has helped me live healthier throughout the years and which I have shared with family and friends. The more you know about eating and drinking healthier, the sooner you will want to change your life and eating habits.

Nutrition is a key part in the process of being healthy and living longer so get started today. The first step is the most important and the most significant.

INTRODUCTION

92 Heartburn Meal and Juice Recipe Solutions: Prevent Heartburn through All Natural Food Sources

By Joe Correa CSN

Heartburn is uncomfortable and never any fun to have but can be easily fixed. This unpleasant condition is actually the return of gastric contents from the stomach into the esophagus and mouth. It is the main symptom of gastroesophageal reflux disease which is why it should be taken seriously.

The decision to pick up this book and finally do something about your heartburn problems is probably the best thing you could have done. Heartburn is the result of have a poor diet, huge amounts of fat, heavy and spicy foods, different 'over the counter' drugs, alcohol, and cigarettes.

This book will solve your problem in a simple but effective manner. It is based on these amazingly delicious recipes that were carefully selected to ease your digestion and prevent gastric contents from returning into your esophagus. This collection of recipes is loaded with proteins, good carbs, vitamins, and minerals.

Start your day with a bowl of cherry oatmeal for an instant energy boost. For lunch, choose an Italian dish 'Cod with Asparagus' which has a mind-blowing source of proteins and antioxidants. When it comes to fats, always make sure you use high-quality olive or coconut oil to give your body a daily dose of precious omega-3 fatty acids. Make sure to especially focus on the most important meal of a day: dinner. People who suffer from heartburn and those who wish to avoid it, must choose to have a light dinner. Physicians and nutritionists agree that a carefully chosen dinner is the best possible way to prevent heartburn.

The meal and juice recipes in this book offer lots of food solutions that will prevent and revert heartburn fast. Try them all and see which ones are your favorite!

92 HEARTBURN MEAL AND JUICE RECIPE SOLUTIONS: PREVENT HEARTBURN THROUGH ALL NATURAL FOOD SOURCES

MEALS

1. Basmati Rice with Carrot

Ingredients:

2 cups of basmati rice, pre-cooked

1 large carrot, grated

3 tbsp of fresh parsley, finely chopped

2 tbsp of balsamic vinegar

2 tbsp of lemon juice, freshly squeezed

½ tsp of Himalayan pink salt

¼ tsp of red pepper flakes

Preparation:

In a small bowl, combine parsley, vinegar, lemon juice, salt, and red pepper. Mix and set aside until you prepare the rice.

In a medium heavy-bottomed, place basmati rice and add about 6 cups of water. Bring it to a boil and then reduce the heat to low. Cover with a lid and cook for 15 minutes. Fluff with a fork and remove from the heat.

Place the rice in a large bowl and add grated carrot. Stir once and then drizzle with the previously prepared dressing. Toss well to coat and serve immediately.

Nutrition information per serving: Kcal: 466, Protein: 9.2g, Carbs: 98g, Fats: 1.1g

2.   Grilled Zucchini with Lemon Dressing

Ingredients:

1 large zucchini, sliced

1 cup of collard greens, chopped

2 tbsp of lemon juice, freshly squeezed

1 tbsp of apple cider vinegar

1 tsbp of extra-virgin olive oil

1 tsp of salt

¼ tsp of black pepper, ground

Preparation:

In a small bowl, combine lemon juice, vinegar, oil, salt, and pepper. Stir well and set aside.

Rinse the collard greens under cold running water. Drain and place in a pot of boiling water. Cook for 2 minutes and remove from the heat. Drain and set aside to cool for a while.

Preheat the grill to a medium-high temperature.

Wash the zucchini and cut into thin slices. Brush the zucchini slices with previously made marinade. Grill for about 3-4 minutes on each side, or until nicely golden brown.

Combine zucchini and collard greens in a serving dish and drizzle with lemon juice dressing. Serve immediately.

Nutrition information per serving: Kcal: 466, Protein: 9.2g, Carbs: 98g, Fats: 1.1g

3.   Cherry Oatmeal

Ingredients:

1 cup of rolled oats

1 cup of coconut milk

4 oz of fresh cherries, pitted and halved

1 medium-sized banana, peeled and chopped

1 tbsp of flaxseeds

1 tbsp of honey

1 cup of water

Preparation:

Pour the water in a medium heavy-bottomed pot. Bring it to a boil and then add oats. Cook for 2 minutes, stirring constantly. Remove from the heat and let it soak for 10 minutes.

Wash the cherries and cut in half. Remove the pits and set aside.

Now, combine oats, milk, cherries, banana, and honey in a large bowl. Stir well to blend and sprinkle with flaxseeds.

Serve immediately.

Nutrition information per serving: Kcal: 399, Protein: 6.4g, Carbs: 48.9g, Fats: 21.7g

4.   Cod with Asparagus

Ingredients:

1 lb of cod fillets

1 cup of fresh asparagus, trimmed

1 tbsp of olive oil

2 tbsp of lemon juice, freshly squeezed

1 tbsp of parsley, finely chopped

2 garlic cloves, crushed

1 tsp of salt

¼ tsp of black pepper, ground

Preparation:

In a small bowl, combine oil, lemon juice, parsley, garlic, salt, and pepper. Stir well to blend and set aside.

Wash the aspargus and trim off the woody ends. Cut into bite-sized pieces and place in a deep pot. Add 2 cups of water and sprinkle with a pinch of salt. Bring it to a boil and then reduce the heat to low. Cook for 10 minutes and remove from the heat. Drain and set aside.

Preheat the grill to medium-high temperature. Generously brush the fillets and gril for about 3-5 minutes on each side. Add more marinade while grilling.

Serve the fillets with asparagus and drizzle with more marinade.

Enjoy!

Nutrition information per serving: Kcal: 214, Protein: 35.8g, Carbs: 2.8g, Fats: 6.1g

5. Veal and Green Bean Stew

Ingredients:

1 lb of lean veal, cut into bite-sized pieces

1 cup of green beans, chopped

1 small onion, chopped

1 cup of tomatoes, diced

1 cup of sweet potatoes, chopped

2 tbsp of olive oil

1 tsp of cayenne pepper

½ tsp of dried oregano, ground

1 tsp of salt

¼ tsp of red pepper, ground

Preparation:

Wash the meat under cold running water and pat dry with a kitchen paper. Cut into bite-sized pieces and set aside.

Preheat the oil in a large deep pot over a medium-high temperature. add meat chops and sprinkle with some salt and cook for 10 minutes, stirring occasionally.

Now, add chopped and prepared vegetables. Pour 4 cups of water and bring it to a boil. Sprinkle with cayenne pepper, oregano, salt, and red pepper. You can add some flour to thicken. However, this is optional. When boiled, reduce the heat to low and cover with a lid. Cook for 30 minutes, or until vegetables tender.

Remove from the heat and serve warm.

Nutrition information per serving: Kcal: 262, Protein: 23.5g, Carbs: 13.4g, Fats: 12.7g

6.   Sesame Muffins

Ingredients:

1 cup of cornmeal

1 cup of buckwheat flour

1 tsp of baking soda

1 tsp of baking powder

1 tbsp of sesame seeds

¼ tsp of salt

½ cup of applesauce

3 tbsp of honey

1 cup of skim milk

Preparation:

Preheat the oven to 375°F.

In a medium bowl, combine milk and sesame seeds. Set aside and let it soak for 10 minutes.

In a large bowl, combine buckwheat flour, baking soda, baking powder, salt, and cornmeal. Stir until combined and then pour the applesauce and honey. Using a hand mixer, blend until well incorporated. Add milk and sesame seeds mixture and blend again for 2 minutes.

Place muffin papers into muffing molds.Spoon the mixture into muffin molds. Place it in the oven and bake for about 15-20 minutes, or until golden brown.

Remove from the oven and let it cool for while before serving.

Nutrition information per serving: Kcal: 206, Protein: 5.8g, Carbs: 43.4g, Fats: 2.1g

7.   Beans & Peas Stew

Ingredients:

1 cup of kidney beans, soaked overnight

1 cup of green peas

1 cup of beef broth

2 cups of water

2 tbsp of all-purpose flour

1 tsp of cayenne pepper, ground

1 large onion, sliced

2 garlic cloves, crushed

½ tsp of cumin, ground

1 tsp of salt

½ tsp of black pepper, ground

1 tsp of olive oil

Preparation:

Soak the beans overnight. Drain and rinse well. Place in a deep pot along with green peas. Bring it to a boil and then cook for 15 minutes. Remove from the heat and drain well. Set aside.

Now, preheat the oil in large deep pot over a medium-high temperature. Add onions and garlic. Stir-fry for about 3-4 minutes, or until translucent. Pour the broth and water. Add beans and peas and bring it all to a boil. Reduce the heat to low and season with cumin, cayenne, salt, and pepper. Cover with a lid and cook for 40 minutes. Stir in the flour and cook for 2 more minutes.

Remove from the heat and give it a good stir before serving. You can add a bayleaf 10 minutes before done for some extra taste. However, this is optional.

Nutrition information per serving: Kcal: 159, Protein: 9.7g, Carbs: 27.3g, Fats: 1.6g

8. Mushroom Lentils

Ingredients:

1 cup of lentils, soaked overnight

1 cup of button mushrooms, chopped

1 small onion, chopped

2 garlic cloves, crushed

¼ cup of celery, sliced

2 tbsp of fresh parsley, finely chopped

2 tbsp of olive oil

3 cups of chicken broth

1 cup of water

Preparation:

Soak the lentils overnight. Place the lentils in a colander and drain. Rinse under cold running water. Transfer to a deep pot and add chicken broth and mushrooms. Bring it to a boil and then cook for 10 minutes. Reduce the heat to low and simmer for 15 more minutes.

Meanwhile, preheat the oil in a medium saucepan over a medium-high temperature. Add onions and celery. Cook for about 3-4 minutes, or until onions translucent. transfer all to a pot and stir well.

Add water and cook for 15 minutes. Remove from the heat and sprinkle with parsley before serving.

Enjoy!

Nutrition information per serving: Kcal: 182, Protein: 11.3g, Carbs: 21.7g, Fats: 5.8g

9.   Collard Greens Tomato Smoothie

Ingredients:

1 cup of collard greens, torn

1 cup of tomatoes, chopped

1 cup of water

1 large lemon, peeled

½ tsp of dried oregano, ground

¼ tsp of turmeric, ground

Preparation:

Using a colander, wash the collard greens under cold running water. Torn with hands and place it in a food processor.

Wash 2 medium-sized tomatoes and place in a bowl. Cut into small pieces and reserve the tomato juice while cutting. Transfer the tomatoes to a food processor along with juices.

Peel the lemon and cut lengthwise in half. Add it to the food processor along with oregano, turmeric and water. Process until all well combined and smooth.

Transfer to serving glasses and add few ice cubes before serving.

Enjoy!

Nutrition information per serving: Kcal: 77, Protein: 5.6g, Carbs: 13.7g, Fats: 10.5g

10.   Crispy Trout Fillets

Ingredients:

1 lb of trout fillets

1 tbsp of olive oil

1 tbsp of Dijon mustard

1 cup of cornstarch

2 large eggs

1 tsp of salt

½ tsp of black pepper, ground

2 tbsp of lemon juice, freshly squeezed

Preparation:

Wash the fillets under cold running water and pat dry with a kitchen paper. Set aside.

Preheat the grill to a medium-high temperature.

In a large bowl, combine cornstarch, mustard, salt, and pepper.

Crack the eggs on a large baking sheet. First, dip the fillets in eggs, then roll out in cornstarch mixture.

Grill the fillets for about 3-5 minutes on both sides, or until nicely crisp. Drizzle the fillets just before set and remove from the grill.

Serve immediately.

Nutrition information per serving: Kcal: 408, Protein: 33.7g, Carbs: 29.9g, Fats: 15.8g

11.   Turkey Breast in Sweet Sauce

Ingredients:

1 lb of turkey breasts, cut into bite-sized pieces

1 tsp of dried thyme, ground

2 tbsp of olive oil

¼ tsp of cumin, ground

3 tbsp of liquid honey

½ tsp of salt

¼ tsp of black pepper, ground

Preparation:

Wash the meat under cold running water and pat dry with a kitchen paper. Cut into bite-sized pieces and set aside.

In a small bowl, combine oil, thyme, cumin, liquid honey, salt, and pepper. Stir until well incorporated and set aside for 10 minutes to allow flavors to meld.

Preheat the oil in a large skillet over a medium-high temperature. Add meat and cook for about 6-7 minutes, or until almost done. Pour in the previously prepared sauce and stir well to combine. Cook for 2 more minutes, or until the meat is golden brown.

Remove from the heat and serve with some fresh vegetables.

Nutrition information per serving: Kcal: 303, Protein: 25.9g, Carbs: 24.1g, Fats: 11.9g

12.   Kale Beet Salad

Ingredients:

1 cup of fresh kale, torn

1 cup of beets, trimmed and chopped

1 large apple, cored, and chopped

4 tbsp of orange juice, freshly squeezed

2 tbsp of lemon juice, freshly squeezed

1 tsp of apple cider vinegar

1 tsp of salt

¼ tsp of cayenne pepper, ground

Preparation:

In a small bowl, combine orange juice, lemon juice, apple cider vinegar, salt, and cayenne pepper. Stir well and set aside for 10 minutes to allow flavors to mingle.

Wash the kale thoroughly under cold running water. Drain and torn with hands. Set aside.

Wash the beets and trim off the green parts. Cut into bite-sized pieces and set aside.

Wash the apple and remove the core. Cut into bite-sized pieces and set aside.

In a large bowl, combine kale, beets, and apple. Drizzle with previously prepared marinade and refrigerate for about 10-15 minutes before serving.

Nutrition information per serving: Kcal: 131, Protein: 3.1g, Carbs: 31.1g, Fats: 0.6g

13.   Stewed Chicken and Veggies

Ingredients:

1 lb of chicken breasts, skinless and boneless

1 large yellow bell pepper, seeded and chopped

1 large green bell pepper, seeded and chopped

3 garlic cloves, minced

1 cup of tomatoes, diced

1 tsp of dried thyme, ground

1 tbsp of olive oil

1 tsp of salt

¼ tsp of red pepper flakes

3 cups of water

Preparation:

Wash the meat under cold running water and pat dry with a kitchen paper. Cut into bite-sized pieces and set aside.

Wash the bell peppers and cut in half. Remove the seeds and chop into small pieces. Set aside.

Preheat the oil in a deep pot over a medium-high temperature. Add meat and cook for about 3-5 minutes, or until slightly browned. Add the tomatoes and water. Bring it to a boil and then reduce the heat to low. Cook for 30 minutes and sprinkle with thyme, salt, and pepper. Cook for 30 minutes, or until set.

Remove from the heat and serve.

Nutrition information per serving: Kcal: 277, Protein: 34g, Carbs: 7.2g, Fats: 12.2g

14.   Fruit Porridge

Ingredients:

1 cup of fresh strawberries, chopped

2 large bananas, peeled and chopped

3 tbsp of walnuts, roughly chopped

¼ tsp of cinnamon

½ cup of coconut milk

1 tsp of vanilla extract

Preparation:

Wash the strawberries under cold running water. Drain and cut into bite-sized pieces. place in a large bowl and set aside.

Peel the bananas and cut into thin slices. Add it to the food processor and blend until smooth. Transfer to a bowl and stir in the coconut milk, cinnamon, and vanilla extract. Top with walnuts and refrigerate for 15 minutes before serving.

Enjoy!

Nutrition information per serving: Kcal: 241, Protein: 4.1g, Carbs: 27.7g, Fats: 14.6g

15.   Quinoa with Carrots and Tomatoes

Ingredients:

1 cup of quinoa

1 large carrot, sliced

2 small tomatoes, chopped

1 small onion, sliced

1 tsp of salt

1 tbsp of olive oil

2 tbsp of lemon juice, freshly squeezed

1 tsp of apple cider vinegar

½ tsp of black pepper, ground

Preparation:

In a small bowl, combine lemon juice, apple cider vinegar, salt, and pepper. Stir until well incorporated and set aside.

Place quinoa in a heavy-bottomed pot. Add 2 cups of water and bring it to a boil. Reduce the heat to low and cover with a lid. Cook for 15 minutes and remove from the heat. Using a colander, drain well and set aside.

In a large salad bowl, combine tomatoes, carrot, onion, and quinoa. Drizzle with previously made dressing and toss well to coat all the ingredients.

Serve immediately.

Nutrition information per serving: Kcal: 282, Protein: 9.1g, Carbs: 43.7g, Fats: 8.3g

16.   Iceberg Orange Salad

Ingredients:

2 large oranges, peeled

1 cup of Iceberg lettuce, roughly chopped

1 large Granny Smith's apple, cored and chopped

2 oz of dried cranberries

3 tbsp of lemon juice, freshly squeezed

1 tbsp of liquid honey

¼ tsp of red pepper flakes

Preparation:

In a small mixing bowl, combine lemon juice and honey. Stir and set aside.

Wash the lettuce thoroughly under cold running water and roughly chop it. Place the salad in a large salad bowl and set aside.

Wash the apple and cut in half. Remove the core and cut into bite-sized pieces. Add it to the bowl with salad.

Peel the oranges and divide into wedges. Cut the wedges in half and add it to the bowl. Stir in the cranberries and drizzle all with previously prepared dressing. Toss well to coat all the ingredients. Refrigerate for 30 minutes before serving.

Enjoy!

Nutrition information per serving: Kcal: 135, Protein: 1.6g, Carbs: 33.1g, Fats: 0.5g

17.   Milky Chicken Wings

Ingredients:

2 lbs of chicken wings

2 tbsp of olive oil

1 tbsp of all-purpose flour

1 tsp of cayenne pepper, ground

1 tsp of dried oregano, ground

3 tbsp of lemon juice, freshly squeezed

½ cup of milk

½ cup of water

1 tsp of yellow mustard

1 tsp of salt

¼ tsp of black pepper, ground

Preparation:

Wash the wings under cold running water and pat dry with a kitchen paper. Set aside.

In a small bowl, combine milk, water, mustard, salt, pepper, lemon juice, and oregano. Mix until well incorporated and set aside.

Preheat the oil in a large skillet over a medium-high temperature. Cook for about 3-5 minutes, or until slightly browned. Pour the previously prepared sauce and reduce the heat to low. Cook for 10 minutes and then remove from the heat.

Serve warm.

Nutrition information per serving: Kcal: 416, Protein: 53.6g, Carbs: 3.1g, Fats: 19.8g

18.   Beef & Mushrooms in Tomato Sauce

Ingredients:

1 lb of lean beef, cut into bite-sized pieces

½ cup of button mushrooms, chopped

1 cup of tomatoes, chopped

2 tbsp of olive oil

1 tbsp of fresh parsley, finely chopped

2 garlic cloves, crushed

1 small red onion, sliced

1 tsp of salt

¼ tsp of black pepper, ground

Preparation:

Wash the meat under cold running water and pat dry with a kitchen paper. Cut into bite-sized pieces and set aside.

Combine tomatoes, garlic, parsley, onion, salt, and pepper in a blender. Process until well pureed and set aside.

Preheat the oil in a large skillet over a medium-high temperature. Add meat and cook for 3 minutes and then add mushrooms. Cook for another 3 minutes, or until meat turns golden brown. Stir occasionally.

Now, pour the tomato puree and stir well to coat the meat. Add about ½ cup of water to adjust the thickness of the sauce. Stir and cook for 5-7 minutes, or until nicely incorporated.

Remove from the heat and serve warm.

Nutrition information per serving: Kcal: 387, Protein: 47.2g, Carbs: 5.8g, Fats: 19g

19.   Grilled Tuna and Zucchini

Ingredients:

1 lb of tuna steaks, skinless and boneless

1 large zucchini, peeled and cubed

2 tbsp of olive oil

2 tbsp of lemon juice, freshly squeezed

1 tbsp of apple cider vinegar

1 tsp of salt

1 tsp od dried rosemary, ground

¼ tsp of black pepper, ground

Preparation:

Wash the steaks under cold running water and pat dry with a kitchen paper. Set aside.

Peel the zucchini and cut into thin slices. Set aside.

In a small bowl, combine oil, lemon juice, vinegar, salt, rosemary, and pepper. Mix until well incorporated and set aside.

Preheat the grill to a medium-high temperature. Generously brush the steaks and zucchini slices with previously prepared marinade. Grill the meat for about 4 minutes on each side, or until desired doneness. Grill the zucchinis about 3 minutes on each side, or until tender.

Remove from the grill and add more marinade before serving.

Enjoy!

Nutrition information per serving: Kcal: 286, Protein: 35g, Carbs: 3.2g, Fats: 14.4g

20. Broccoli Soup

Ingredients:

1 lb of fresh broccoli, chopped

2 cups of chicken broth

1 cup of skim milk

1 tbsp of butter

1 tsp of cayenne pepper, ground

1 tbsp of fresh parsley, finely chopped

1 tsp of salt

¼ tsp of black pepper, ground

Preparation:

Wash the broccoli under cold running water. Drain and cut into bite-sized pieces. Set aside.

Place the broccoli, chicken broth, and water in a deep saucepan. Bring it to a boil and then reduce the heat to low. Cook for 10 minutes.

Meanwhile, melt the butter in a frying pan over a medium-high temperature. stir in the cayenne pepper and flour. Cook for 1 minute, until nicely blended and creamy.

Remove from the heat and pour into the saucepan. Stir until well incorporated and cook for 3 more minutes.

Remove from the heat and serve warm.

Nutrition information per serving: Kcal: 72, Protein: 5.2g, Carbs: 7.6g, Fats: 2.7g

21.   Onion Parsley Omelet

Ingredients:

5 large eggs, beaten

1 tbsp of fresh parsley, finely chopped

1 small onion, sliced

1 tbsp of olive oil

½ tsp of salt

¼ tsp of cayenne pepper, ground

Preparation:

In a large bowl, whisk the eggs, parsley, salt, and cayenne pepper. Set aside.

Preheat the oil in a large frying pan over a medium-high temperature. Add onions and stir-fry for about 3-4 minutes, or until translucent. Using a wooden spatula, move the onions to one side of the pan.

Now, pour the egg mixture and cook for 3 minutes, and then flip the omelet. Cook for 2 more minutes and fold the omelet.

Remove from the heat and serve immediately.

Nutrition information per serving: Kcal: 254, Protein: 16.2g, Carbs: 4.5g, Fats: 19.5g

22.   Peach Strawberry Smoothie

Ingredients:

1 cup of strawberries, chopped

1 large peach, pitted and chopped

1 large banana, sliced

1 cup of skim milk

1 tbsp of chia seeds

Preparation:

Using a colander, wash the strawberries under cold running water. Drain and chop into small pieces. Add it to the food processor.

Wash the peach and cut in half. Remove the pit cut into bite-sized pieces. Add it to the food processor along with milk and chopped banana. Process until creamy and smooth. Transfer to serving glasses and refrigerate for 15 minutes. Garnish with mint before serving.

Nutrition information per serving: Kcal: 157, Protein: 6.1g, Carbs: 26.2g, Fats: 3.6g

23. Mussels in Tomato Sauce

Ingredients:

1 lb of mussels, shelled

1 medium-sized onion, chopped

1 cup of tomatoes, diced

2 tbsp of tomato paste

2 tbsp of fresh parsley, finely chopped

1 tsp of dried oregano, ground

2 garlic cloves, minced

1 tsp of sea salt

¼ tsp of black pepper, ground

2 tbsp of olive oil

Preparation:

Preheat the oil in a large skillet over a medium-high temperature. Add onions and garlic and cook for 3 minutes, or until slightly translucent. Add mussels and stir in the tomatoes and tomato paste. Add ½ cup of water and stir well to combine. Bring it to a boil and then reduce the heat to low.

Simmer for 10 minutes and stir in the parsley, oregano, salt, and pepper. Stir well and cook for 2 minutes.

Remove from the heat and serve immediately.

Nutrition information per serving: Kcal: 188, Protein: 14.8g, Carbs: 11g, Fats: 9.8g

24.   Sea Bass with Fresh Salad

Ingredients:

1 lb of sea bass fillets

1 cup of Romaine lettuce

1 medium-sized tomato

1 small onion, chopped

2 garlic cloves, crushed

2 tbsp of lemon juice, freshly squeezed

1 tsp of apple cider vinegar

2 tbsp of olive oil

1 tbsp of fresh rosemary, finely chopped

1 tsp of sea salt

¼ tsp of black pepper, ground

Preparation:

Wash the fillets under cold running water and pat dry with a kitchen paper. Cut into thin slices and set aside.

In a small bowl, combine lemon juice, vinegar, rosemary, salt, and pepper. Stir well to mix and set aside to allow flavors to mingle.

Preheat the oil in a large skillet over a medium-high temperature. Add garlic and onion and stir-fry for 2 minutes. Add fillets and cook for about 3-4 minutes on each side. Remove from the heat and transfer to a serving dish.

Wash the lettuce thoroughly and roughly chop it. Wash the tomatoes and cut into bite-sized pieces. Combine with lettuce and drizzle with previously prepared dressing.

Serve fillets with fresh salad.

Nutrition information per serving: Kcal: 297, Protein: 36.7g, Carbs: 6g, Fats: 13.6g

25. Chicken in Cream Tomato Sauce

Ingredients:

1 lb of chicken breasts, skinless and boneless

1 tbsp of lemon juice, freshly squeezed

1 small red onion, sliced

2 garlic cloves, crushed

1 tbsp of olive oil

¼ cup of cream cheese

1 large tomato, diced

1 tsp of dried oregano, ground

1 tsp of sea salt

¼ tsp of black pepper, ground

Preparation:

Wash the meat under cold running water and pat dry with a kitchen paper. Set aside.

Combine tomato, cream cheese, garlic, dried tomato, sea salt, and pepper in food processor or a blender. Process until nicely smooth and creamy. Set aside.

Preheat the oil in a large skillet over a medium-high temperature. Add onions and stir-fry for 3 minutes. Add meat and cook for 5 minutes, stirring occasionally.

Pour the previously prepared sauce and cook until heated trough. Reduce the heat to low and cook for 2 more minutes. Remove from the heat and serve.

Nutrition information per serving: Kcal: 316, Protein: 34.7g, Carbs: 4.7g, Fats: 17.2g

26.   Brussels Sprouts with Onions

Ingredients:

1 lb of fresh Brussels sprouts, chopped

2 large onions, sliced

2 garlic cloves, crushed

2 tbsp of olive oil

1 tsp of salt

¼ tsp of black pepper, ground

1 tbsp of all-purpose flour

1 tsp of cayenne pepper

1 tbsp of tomato paste

¼ tsp of dried rosemary, ground

Preparation:

Wash the Brussels sprouts under cold running water and trim off the outer wilted layers. Cut into bite-sized pieces and set aside.

In a small bowl, combine tomato paste, rosemary, flour and 2 tablespoons of water. Stir until well incorporated and set aside.

Preheat the oil in large saucepan over a medium-high temperature. Add onions and stir-fry for about 4-5 minutes or until translucent. Add Brussels sprouts and about ½ cup of water. Bring it to a boil and cook for 5 minutes, or until water almost evaporates. Stir in the tomato paste mixture and reduce the heat to low. Cook for 4 more minutes and remove from the heat.

Serve warm.

Nutrition information per serving: Kcal: 143, Protein: 4.5g, Carbs: 17.7g, Fats: 7.6g

27.   Mackerel with Avocado Puree

Ingredients:

1 lb of mackerel fillets

1 medium-sized avocado, pitted and chopped

1 small onion, chopped

1 medium-sized tomato, chopped

2 garlic cloves, crushed

1 tsp of dried oregano, ground

1 tbsp of lemon juice, freshly squeezed

1 tbsp of olive oil

1 tsp of salt

¼ tsp of black pepper, freshly ground

Preparation:

Wash the fillets under cold running water and pat dry with a kitchen paper. Set aside.

In a food processor, combine avocado, onion, tomato, garlic,oregano, salt, and pepper. Process until creamy and set aside.

Preheat the oil in a large nonstick skillet over a medium-high temperature. Add fillets and cook for 3 minutes on each side, or until set.

Remove from the heat and sprinkle with lemon juice. Serve with avocado puree.

Nutrition information per serving: Kcal: 447, Protein: 28.6g, Carbs: 8.1g Fats: 33.7g

28.   Orange Cream Smoothie

Ingredients:

2 large oranges, peeled and wedged

1 medium-sized carrot

½ tsp of turmeric, ground

½ cup of sour cream

2 tbsp of skim milk

¼ tsp of cinnamon, ground

1 tbsp of fresh mint, chopped

Preparation:

Wash the carrots and remove the green parts. Remove the top od each carrot and slice them. Peel the oranges and divide into wedges.

Now, combine orange, carrot, milk, and sour cream in a food processor. Process until creamy and smooth. Transfer to serving glasses and stir in the turmeric and cinnamon. Garnish with mint and refrigerate for 15 minutes before serving.

Nutrition information per serving: Kcal: 154, Protein: 3g, Carbs: 19.1g Fats: 8.2g

29.   Beef Potato Casserole

Ingredients:

1 lb of lean ground beef

1 cup of green beans

1 large potato, peeled sliced

1 medium-sized onion

2 tbsp of buckwheat flour

2 tbsp of fresh parsley, finely chopped

1 tsp of salt

¼ tsp of red pepper, ground

1 tbsp of olive oil

Preparation:

Preheat the oven to 375°F.

Place the green beans in a pot of boiling water and cook for 5 minutes. Remove from the heat and drain well. Set aside.

Peel the potato and cut into thin slices. Place in a deep pot and add 3 cups of water. Bring it to a boil and then cook for

10 minutes. Remove from the heat and drain well. Set aside to cool for a while.

Meanwhile, combine ground beef, flour, green beans, parsley, salt, and pepper in a large bowl.

Grease a large casserole dish with some oil. Spread the potatoes on the bottom of the dish. Top with beef mixture and spread evenly. Place it in the oven and bake for about 45-50 minutes, or until doneness.

Remove from the oven and let cool for a while before cutting and serving.

Nutrition information per serving: Kcal: 277, Protein: 30.1g, Carbs: 19.2g Fats: 8.7g

30.   Apricots in Coconut Cream

Ingredients:

4 medium-sized apricots

1 large banana, sliced

3 tbsp of coconut milk

1 tbsp of honey

1 tsp of vanilla extract

½ cup of sour cream

1 tbsp of orange juice, freshly squeezed

Preparation:

Wash the apricots and cut in half. Remove the pits and cut into bite-sized pieces. Set aside,

Peel the banana and cut into thin slices.

Now, pour the coconut milk in a small saucepan. Heat up to a medium heat and stir in the honey. Reduce the heat to low and add vanilla extract, stirring constantly. Cook for 1 minute and then add sour cream. Stir well and cook until heated trough and creamy. Remove from the heat and stir in the orange juice.

Combine apricots and banana in a bowl and pour the cream. Toss well to coat all the ingredients. Set aside to cool to a room temperature and then refrigerate for 30 minutes before serving.

Enjoy!

Nutrition information per serving: Kcal: 310, Protein: 4.1g, Carbs: 36.7g Fats: 18.1g

31.   Cranberry Tuna Steaks

Ingredients:

1 lb of tuna steaks

1 cup of cranberries

3 tbsp of skim milk

1 tbsp of honey

2 tbsp of olive oil

1 tbsp of apple cider vinegar

1 tsp of dried thyme, ground

2 tbsp of lemon juice, freshly squeezed

1 tsp sea salt

¼ tsp of black pepper, freshly ground

Preparation:

In a small saucepan, heat up the milk, honey, and cranberries over a medium-high temperature. cook until heat trough and mixture turns to creamy and jelly.

Remove from the heat and set aside.

Preheat the oil in a large skillet over a medium-high temperature. Add steaks and cook for 3 minutes. Turn the steaks and add vinegar and lemon juice. Cook for 3 minutes more, or until doneness.

Remove from the heat and sprinkle with thyme, salt, and pepper to taste. Serve with cranberry sauce.

Enjoy!

Nutrition information per serving: Kcal: 410, Protein: 45.9g, Carbs: 10.4g Fats: 18.9g

32.   Cream Asparagus Soup

Ingredients:

1 lb of asparagus, trimmed and chopped

1 cup of skim milk

1 cup of chicken broth

2 tbsp of all-purpose flour

1 tsp of dried oregano, ground

1 tsp of salt

¼ tsp of black pepper, ground

Preparation:

Wash the asparagus and trim off the woody ends. Cut into bite-sized pieces and place them in a large saucepan. Pour the milk and cook until heated trough. Add chicken broth and stir well. Bring it to a boil and then reduce the heat to low.

Stir in the flour, oregano, salt, and pepper. Cook for 5 more minutes, or until the asparagus tender.

Remove from the heat and serve warm.

Nutrition information per serving: Kcal: 56, Protein: 4.9g, Carbs: 8.8g Fats: 0.4g

33. Spring Onion Tomato Omelet

Ingredients:

5 large eggs, beaten

1 small tomato, chopped

½ cup of spring onions, chopped

1 tbsp of fresh parsley, finely chopped

¼ tsp of red pepper flakes

1 tsp of Himalayan pink salt

1 tbsp of olive oil

Preparation:

In a large bowl, whisk the eggs, parsley, red pepper, and salt. Set aside.

Preheat the oil in a large skillet over a medium-high temperature. Add spring onions and cook for 1 minutes, stirring constantly. Add tomatoes and cook for another minute, until combined with onions.

Pour the egg mixture and spread evenly in the skillet. Cook for about 3 minutes then flip the omelet. Cook for 1 minute more, or until eggs are set.

Remove from the heat and fold the omelet. Serve immediately.

Nutrition information per serving: Kcal: 256, Protein: 16.7g, Carbs: 4.8g Fats: 19.6g

34.   Chia Oats with Cinnamon

Ingredients:

2 cups of skim milk

1 cup of rolled oats

1 tbsp of chia seeds

2 large egg whites

1 tbsp of honey

1 tsp of cinnamon, ground

Preparation:

Pour the milk in a heavy-bottomed pot. Bring it to a boil and then reduce the heat to low.

Add oats, egg whites, and cinnamon. Stir until well incorporated and cook for about 5-7 minutes. Remove from the heat and stir in the chia seeds. Set aside to cool for a while before serving.

You can stir in some dried or fresh fruits. However, this is optional.

Enjoy!

Nutrition information per serving: Kcal: 208, Protein: 11.9g, Carbs: 34g Fats: 2.7g

35.   Pepper Salmon Pate

Ingredients:

1 lb of salmon fillets

1 medium-sized red bell pepper, seeded and chopped

1 small onion, chopped

1 tbsp of yellow mustard

1 tsp of balsamic vinegar

1 tsp of dried rosemary, ground

1 tsp of sea salt

¼ tsp of black pepper, freshly ground

1 tbsp of lemon juice, freshly squeezed

1 tbsp of olive oil

Preparation:

Wash the fillets under cold running water and pat dry with a kitchen paper. Cut into bite-sized pieces and set aside.

Preheat the oil in a large skillet over a medium-high temperature. Add onions and stir-fry for 3 minutes. Add tuna chops and cook for 6-8 minutes, stirring constantly.

Sprinkle with some salt and give it a good stir. Remove from the heat and transfer all to a food processor.

Add all remaining ingredients to a food processor and blend until creamy and pureed.

Transfer to a bowl and serve immediately.

Nutrition information per serving: Kcal: 269, Protein: 30.3g, Carbs: 6g Fats: 14.4g

36.   Kale Muffins

Ingredients:

¼ cup of fresh kale, finely chopped

2 cups of buckwheat flour

1 tsp of baking powder

1 cup of low-fat milk

2 large eggs

4 tbsp of cream cheese

1 tbsp of vegetable oil

Preparation:

Preheat the oven to 300°F.

Wash the kale thoroughly under cold running water. Drain and finely chop it and set aside.

In a large bowl, combine flour and baking powder and stir well. Set aside.

In a separate large bowl, combine milk, eggs, cream, and vegetable oil. Using a hand mixer, blend until well incorporated. Now, pour this mixture into a bowl with flour and blend on low speed until you get a nice dough.

Place some muffin papers in a muffin molds. Spoon the dough into muffin molds and place it in the oven.

Bake for about 20-25 minutes, or until golden brown. Remove from the oven and set aside to cool for a while.

Enjoy!

Nutrition information per serving: Kcal: 441, Protein: 18.2g, Carbs: 62.5g Fats: 15.8g

37.   Onion Creamy Chicken

Ingredients:

1 lb of chicken breasts, skinless and boneless

1 large onion, sliced

1 tbsp of olive oil

2 garlic cloves, crushed

2 tbsp sour cream

2 tbsp of fresh parsley, finely chopped

1 tsp of salt

¼ tsp of black pepper, ground

Preparation:

Wash the chicken breasts under cold running water and pat dry with a kitchen paper. Cut into 1-inch thick pieces and set aside.

In a small bowl, combine sour cream, parsley, garlic, salt, and pepper. Stir well and set aside.

Preheat the oil in a large skillet over a medium-high temperature. Add onions and stir-fry for about 3-4 minutes, or until translucent. Add chicken chops and cook for 10 minutes, or until nicely golden. Pour over the previously prepared sauce and stir well to coat the chicken.

Cook for 2 more minutes and remove from the heat. Set aside to cool for a while before serving.

Enjoy!

Nutrition information per serving: Kcal: 369, Protein: 44.8g, Carbs: 6g Fats: 17.6g

38. Navy Bean Salad

Ingredients:

1 cup of navy beans, pre-cooked

1 cup Iceberg lettuce, chopped

1 medium-sized tomato, chopped

1 medium-sized yellow bell pepper, chopped

1 small red onion, chopped

2 tbsp of lemon juice, freshly squeezed

1 tsp of balsamic vinegar

1 tbsp of fresh parsley, finely chopped

2 tbsp of olive oil

2 garlic cloves, minced

1 tsp of salt

¼ tsp of red pepper flakes

Preparation:

In a small bowl, combine lemon juice, vinegar, parsley, olive oil, garlic, salt, and pepper. Stir until well incorporated and set aside for 15 minutes to allow flavors to meld.

Soak the beans overnight. Drain and rinse well. Place the beans in a deep pot and add 3 cups of water. Bring it to a boil and then cook for 10 minutes, or until tender. Remove from the heat and drain well. Set aside.

Wash and prepare the vegetables. Cut the pepper in half and remove the seeds. Chop into small pieces. Set aside.

Peel the onion and roughly chop it. Cut the tomato in small pieces and set aside.

In a large salad bowl, combine tomato, bell pepper, and onion. Stir once and then add beans. Drizzle with previously prepared dressing and give it a good stir.

Make a layer of lettuce on a serving plate. Spoon the salad onto it and serve immediately.

Nutrition information per serving: Kcal: 352, Protein: 16.9g, Carbs: 50.5g Fats: 10.7g

39.   Turkey with Ginger Sauce

Ingredients:

1 lb of turkey fillets

1 tbsp of olive oil

1 tbsp of fresh parsley, finely chopped

1 small onion, finely chopped

1 ginger root knob, 1-inch thick

2 garlic cloves, crushed

1 tsp of apple cider vinegar

1 tbsp of lemon juice, freshly squeezed

1 tsp of salt

¼ tsp of black pepper

Preparation:

Peel the ginger root knob and place it in a food processor along with onion, garlic, vinegar, and lemon juice. Process until creamy and smooth. Set aside.

Preheat the oil in a large saucepan over a medium-high temperature. Add turkey chops and cook for about 8-10 minutes, or until nicely golden brown. Sprinkle with parsley, salt, and pepper to taste. Stir once and then remove from the heat.

Serve the meat with ginger sauce.

Nutrition information per serving: Kcal: 318, Protein: 44.9g, Carbs: 4.4g Fats: 12.4g

40.   Salted Tomato Beet Smoothie

Ingredients:

1 large tomato, chopped

1 small cucumber, chopped

1 medium-sized beet, trimmed and chopped

1 cup of Greek yogurt

½ tsp of salt

½ tsp of apple cider vinegar

¼ tsp of red pepper, ground

Preparation:

Wash the tomato and place in a bowl. Cut into bite-sized pieces and reserve the tomato juice while cutting. Transfer the tomato and juice to a food processor. Set aside.

Wash the cucumber and cut into thin slices. Add it to the food processor and set aside.

Wash the beet and trim off the green parts. Cut into small pieces and add it to the food processor along with yogurt, salt, vinegar, and pepper.

Process until smooth and creamy. Transfer to serving glasses and refrigerate for 10 minutes before serving.

Enjoy!

Nutrition information per serving: Kcal: 81, Protein: 7.8g, Carbs: 10.1g Fats: 1.5g

41.   Cutlets with Basmati Rice

Ingredients:

1 lb of veal cutlets, boneless

1 cup of basmati rice

3 cups of water

2 garlic cloves, crushed

2 tbsp of lemon juice, freshly squeezed

1 tsp of turmeric, ground

1 tsp of dried thyme, ground

1 tbsp of olive oil

1 tsp of salt

¼ tsp of black pepper, freshly ground

Preparation:

Wash the meat under cold running water and pat dry with a kitchen paper. Cut into thin slices and set aside.

Pour the water in a deep pot. bring it to a boil over a medium-high temperature. Add rice and cook for 10 minutes. Reduce the heat to low, and stir in the turmeric.

Stir well to combine and cook for about 4-5 minutes. Remove from the heat and cover with a lid. Set aside.

Preheat the grill to a medium-high temperature.

Meanwhile, combine oil, garlic, thyme, and lemon juice in a small bowl. Stir well and brush the meat with this marinade. Grill for about 4-5 minutes on each side, or until desired doneness. Transfer to serving plates and drizzle with the remaining marinade.

Serve the meat with previously prepared basmati rice.

Nutrition information per serving: Kcal: 267, Protein: 21.5g, Carbs: 21.8g Fats: 9.6g

42. Brown Rice with Stewed Vegetables

Ingredients:

1 cup of brown rice, uncooked

8oz fresh cauliflower

2 medium-sized carrots, sliced

1 medium sized cellery root, sliced

1 tsp of pink Himalayan salt

½ tsp of freshly ground black pepper

2 tbsp of extra coconut oil

1 tablespoon of fresh celery, finely chopped

Preparation:

Place one cup of brown rice in a deep pot. Add three cups of water and bring it to a boil. Reduce the heat and continue to cook until the liquid evaporates. Remove from the heat and set aside.

Meanwhile, boil the vegetables and cook until soft. Remove from the heat and drain.

Melt the coconut oil over a medium-hogh heat. Add cooked rice, salt, pepper and stir-fry for 3-4 minutes. Mix well and serve with sliced vegetables.

Add some chopped celery and serve warm.

Nutrition information per serving: Kcal: 399 Protein: 10g, Carbs: 84.8g, Fats: 2.7g

JUICES

1.   Watermelon Beet Juice

Ingredients:

1 cup of watermelon, cubed

1 whole beet, chopped

1 small Granny Smith's apple, cored

Preparation:

Cut the top of the watermelon. Cut lengthwise in half and then cut one large wedge. Peel it and cut into small cubes. Remove the seeds and fill the measuring cup. Wrap the rest in a plastic foil and refrigerate for later.

Wash and trim off the beet. Cut into bite-sized pieces and set aside.

Wash the apple and cut in half. Remove the core and cut into small pieces. Set aside.

Now, combine watermelon, beet, and apple in a juicer and process until well juiced. Transfer to a serving glass and refrigerate for 15 minutes before serving.

Garnish with mint and enjoy!

Nutrition information per serving: Kcal: 138, Protein: 2.8g, Carbs: 38.9g, Fats: 0.6g

2.   Banana Broccoli Juice

Ingredients:

1 large banana, chunked

2 cups of broccoli, chopped

1 cup of Romaine lettuce, shredded

2 oz of coconut water

Preparation:

Peel the banana and cut into small chunks. Set aside.

Wash the broccoli and trim off the outer wilted layers. Cut into small pieces and fill the measuring cup. Reserve the rest in the refrigerator.

Rinse the lettuce thoroughly under cold running water. Shred it and fill the measuring cup. Reserve the rest for later.

Now, combine banana, broccoli, and lettuce in a juicer and process until juiced. Transfer to a serving glass and stir in the coconut water.

Add some crushed ice and serve immediately.

Nutrition information per serving: Kcal: 153, Protein: 7.2g, Carbs: 44.7g, Fats: 1.3g

3.   Avocado Aloe Juice

Ingredients:

1 cup of avocado, cubed

1 cup of collard greens, chopped

1 cup of fresh mint, chopped

1 large Golden Delicious apple, cored

1 oz of aloe juice

Preparation:

Peel the avocado and cut into half. Remove the pit and cut into small cubes. Fill the measuring cup and reserve the rest for later.

Combine collard greens and mint in a colander. Wash thoroughly under cold running water and slightly drain. Chop all into small pieces and set aside.

Wash the apple and cut in half. Remove the core and cut into bite-sized pieces. Set aside.

Now, combine avocado, collard greens, mint, and apple in a juicer. Process until well juiced. Transfer to a serving glass and stir in the aloe juice.

Refrigerate for 10 minutes before serving.

Nutrition information per serving: Kcal: 318, Protein: 5.6g, Carbs: 47.7g, Fats: 22.7g

4.   Fennel Ginger Juice

Ingredients:

1 medium-sized fennel bulb

1 small ginger knob, peeled

1 medium-sized carrot, sliced

1 large cabbage leaf, torn

Preparation:

Wash the fennel and trim off the green ends. Using a sharp paring knife, remove the outer layer. Cut into small pieces and set aside.

Peel the ginger knob and cut into small pieces. Set aside.

Wash and peel the carrot. Cut into thin slices and set aside.

Wash the cabbage leaf and torn with hands. Set aside.

Now, combine fennel, ginger, carrot, and cabbage in a juicer and process until juiced. Transfer to a serving glass and refrigerate before serving.

Enjoy!

Nutrition information per serving: Kcal: 72, Protein: 4g, Carbs: 25.9g, Fats: 0.7g

5.   Pepper Cauliflower Juice

Ingredients:

1 large red bell pepper, chopped

1 cup of cauliflower, chopped

1 cup of Brussels sprouts, halved

1 oz of water

Preparation:

Wash the bell pepper and cut lengthwise in half. Remove the seeds and the top stem. Cut into small pieces and set aside.

Trim off the outer leaves of a cauliflower. Wash it and cut into small pieces. Fill the measuring cup and reserve the rest in the refrigerator.

Wash the Brussels sprouts and trim off the wilted layers. Cut each in half and fill the measuring cup. Set aside.

Now, combine pepper, cauliflower, and Brussels sprouts in a juicer and process until juiced. Transfer to a serving glass and stir in the water.

Nutrition information per serving: Kcal: 106, Protein: 9.6g, Carbs: 30.9g, Fats: 1.3g

6. Pumpkin Apple Juice

Ingredients:

1 cup of pumpkin, cubed

1 small green apple, cored

1 small pear, chopped

1 small ginger knob, peeled

1 oz of water

Preparation:

Peel the pumpkin and cut lengthwise in half. Scoop out the seeds and cut into small cubes. Fill the measuring cup and reserve the rest in the refrigerator.

Wash the apple and cut in half. Remove the core and cut into bite-sized pieces. Set aside.

Wash the pear and cut in half. Remove the core and cut into small chunks. Set aside.

Peel the ginger and cut into small pieces. Set aside.

Now, combine pumpkin, apple, pear, and ginger in a juicer and process until juiced. Transfer to a serving glass and stir in the water.

Add some ice and serve immediately.

Nutrition information per serving: Kcal: 167, Protein: 2.4g, Carbs: 50.7g, Fats: 0.6g

7.   Celery Asparagus Juice

Ingredients:

1 cup of celery, chopped

1 cup of asparagus, trimmed and chopped

1 large banana, peeled and chunked

1 small ginger knob, 1-inch thick

1 oz. of water

Preparation:

Wash the celery stalks and cut into bite-sized pieces. Fill the measuring cup and reserve the rest for some other juice.

Wash the asparagus and trim off the woody ends. Cut into bite-sized pieces and set aside.

Peel the banana and cut into small chunks. Set aside.

Peel the ginger knob and chop it.

Now, combine celery, asparagus, banana, and ginger in a juicer and process until juiced. Transfer to a serving glass and stir in the water.

Add some crushed ice and serve immediately.

Nutrition information per serving: Kcal: 138, Protein: 5.3g, Carbs: 40.3g, Fats: 0.8g

8.   Cauliflower Carrot Juice

Ingredients:

1 cup of cauliflower, chopped

1 cup of carrots, sliced

1 cup of purple cabbage, chopped

1 cup of collard greens, chopped

Preparation:

Wash the cauliflower and trim off the outer leaves. Cut into bite-sized pieces and fill the measuring cup. Reserve the rest for later.

Wash and peel the carrots. Cut into thin slices and fill the measuring cup. Set aside.

Combine cabbage and collard greens in a colander. Wash thoroughly under cold running water and slightly drain. Chop into small pieces and set aside.

Now, combine cauliflower, carrots, cabbage, and collard greens in a juicer and process until juiced. Transfer to a serving glass and refrigerate for 10 minutes before serving.

Nutrition information per serving: Kcal: 138, Protein: 5.3g, Carbs: 40.3g, Fats: 0.8g

9.   Kale Banana Juice

Ingredients:

1 cup of fresh kale, chopped

1 large banana, peeled and chunked

1 small Granny Smith's apple, cored

1 cup of Brussels sprouts, halved

¼ tsp of ginger, ground

1 oz. of coconut water

Preparation:

Wash the kale thoroughly under cold running water and slightly drain. Chop into small pieces and set aside.

Peel the banana and cut into small chunks. Set aside.

Wash the apple and cut in half. Remove the core and cut into bite-sized pieces. Set aside.

Wash the Brussels sprouts and remove the outer wilted layers. Cut each in half and set aside.

Now, combine kale, banana, apple, and Brussels sprouts in a juicer and process until juiced. Transfer to a serving glass and stir in the coconut water and ginger.

Add some ice and serve immediately.

Nutrition information per serving: Kcal: 223, Protein: 7.9g, Carbs: 64.4g, Fats: 1.6g

10.   Leek Potato Juice

Ingredients:

1 whole leek, chopped

1 cup of sweet potatoes, cubed

1 cup of turnip greens, torn

1 cup of cucumber, sliced

1 large carrot, sliced

¼ tsp of salt

1 oz of water

Preparation:

Wash the leek and cut into bite-sized pieces. Set aside.

Peel the potato and cut into small cubes. Fill the measuring cup and reserve the rest for later.

Place the turnip greens in a colander and rinse under running water. Slightly drain and torn with hands. Set aside.

Peel the cucumber and cut into thin slices. Fill the measuring cup and reserve the rest in the refrigerator.

Wash and peel the carrot. Cut into thin slices and set aside.

Now, combine leek, potato, turnip greens, cucumber, and carrot in a juicer and process until juiced. Transfer to a serving glass and stir in the salt and water.

Serve cold.

Nutrition information per serving: Kcal: 186, Protein: 5.3g, Carbs: 52.1g, Fats: 0.7g

11.   Cauliflower Kale Juice

Ingredients:

2 cups of cauliflower, chopped

1 cup of fresh kale, chopped

1 cup of Romaine lettuce, chopped

1 cup of fresh basil, chopped

1 cup of cucumber, sliced

Preparation:

Wash the cauliflower head and trim off the outer leaves. Wash and chop into bite-sized pieces. Fill the measuring cup and reserve the rest in the refrigerator.

Combine kale, lettuce, and basil in a large colander. Wash thoroughly under cold running water and slightly drain. Chop all into small pieces and set aside.

Wash the cucumber and cut into thin slices. Fill the measuring cup and reserve the rest for later. Set aside.

Now, combine cauliflower, kale, lettuce, basil, and cucumber in a juicer and process until juiced. Transfer to a serving glass and refrigerate for 10 minutes before serving.

Nutrition information per serving: Kcal: 76, Protein: 8.6g, Carbs: 20.6g, Fats: 1.6g

12. Guava Pineapple Juice

Ingredients:

1 whole guava, chopped

1 cup of pineapple, chunked

1 cup of cucumber, sliced

1 cup of fresh mint, torn

1 oz. of water

Preparation:

Wash and peel the guava fruit. Chop into bite-sized pieces and set aside.

Cut the top of the pineapple and peel it using a sharp paring knife. Peel it and cut into small pieces. Set aside.

Wash the cucumber and cut into thin slices. Fill the measuring cup and reserve the rest in the refrigerator.

Wash the mint and slightly drain. Torn with hands and set aside.

Now, combine guava, pineapple, cucumber, and mint in a juicer and process until juiced. Transfer to a serving glass and stir in the water.

Refrigerate for 10 minutes before serving.

Nutrition information per serving: Kcal: 115, Protein: 3.6g, Carbs: 35.2g, Fats: 1.1g

13. Zucchini Pear Juice

Ingredients:

1 small zucchini, sliced

1 medium-sized pear, chopped

1 medium-sized banana, chunked

1 large strawberry, chopped

1 oz. of water

Preparation:

Wash the zucchini and cut into small chunks. Set aside.

Wash the pear and cut in half. Remove the core and cut into bite-sized pieces. Set aside.

Peel the banana and cut into small chunks. Set aside.

Wash the strawberry and remove the stem. Cut into small pieces and set aside.

Now, combine zucchini, pear, banana, and strawberry in a juicer and process until juiced. Transfer to a serving glass and stir in the water.

Add some crushed ice and serve immediately.

Nutrition information per serving: Kcal: 191, Protein: 3.5g, Carbs: 59.1g, Fats: 1.1g

14.   Honeydew Mint Juice

Ingredients:

1 large wedge of honeydew melon, chopped

1 cup of fresh mint, chopped

1 cup of mustard greens, chopped

1 small Granny Smith's apple, cored

1 oz. of water

Preparation:

Cut the melon in half. Cut one large wedge and peel the peel it. Cut into small pieces and set aside. Wrap the rest of the melon in a plastic foil and refrigerate for later.

Combine mint and mustard greens in a colander and wash thoroughly. Slightly drain and chop into small pieces. Set aside.

Wash the apple and cut lengthwise in half. Remove the core and cut into bite-sized pieces. Set aside.

Now, combine melon, mint, mustard greens and apple in a juicer and process until juiced.

Transfer to a serving glass and stir in the water. Refrigerate for 10 minutes before serving.

Nutrition information per serving: Kcal: 139, Protein: 4.1g, Carbs: 40.5g, Fats: 0.9g

15.　Brussels Sprout Pumpkin Juice

Ingredients:

2 cups of Brussels sprouts, halved

1 cup of pumpkin, cubed

2 large carrots, sliced

1 small ginger knob, peeled and chopped

1 oz. of water

Preparation:

Wash the Brussels sprouts and trim off the outer wilted layers. Cut each sprout in half and set aside.

Cut the pumpkin in half and scoop out the seeds. For one cup, you'll need about one large wedge. Cut and peel. Chop into bite-sized pieces and fill the measuring cup. Wrap the rest of the pumpkin in a plastic foil and reserve in the refrigerator.

Wash and peel the carrots. Cut into thin slices and set aside.

Peel the ginger knob and chop it into small pieces. Set aside.

Now, combine Brussels sprouts, pumpkin, carrots, and ginger in a juicer and process until juiced. Transfer to a serving glass and stir in the water.

Add some ice and serve immediately.

Nutrition information per serving: Kcal: 127, Protein: 8.5g, Carbs: 38.2g, Fats: 1.1g

16.   Watermelon Cantaloupe Juice

Ingredients:

1 cup of watermelon, cubed

1 cup of cantaloupe, diced

1 small banana, chunked

¼ tsp of cinnamon, ground

Preparation:

Cut the watermelon lengthwise in half. For one cup, cut one large wedge. Peel and chop into small cubes. Remove the seeds and fill the measuring cup. Reserve the rest in the refrigerator.

Cut the cantaloupe in half and scoop out the seeds. Cut and peel two medium wedges. Fill the measuring cup and reserve the rest for later.

Peel the banana and cut into chunks. Set aside.

Now, combine watermelon, cantaloupe, and banana in a juicer and process until juiced. Transfer to a serving glass and stir in the cinnamon. Refrigerate for 10 minutes before serving.

Enjoy!

Nutrition information per serving: Kcal: 171, Protein: 3.4g, Carbs: 47.3g, Fats: 0.8g

17.   Potato Cabbage Juice

Ingredients:

1 cup of sweet potatoes, cubed

1 medium-sized artichoke, chopped

1 cup of cucumber, sliced

1 cup of green cabbage, chopped

Preparation:

Peel the sweet potato and cut into small cubes. Fill the measuring cup and reserve the rest for some other juice. Set aside.

Using a sharp paring knife, peel the artichoke and cut into bite-sized pieces. Set aside.

Wash the cucumber and cut into thin slices. fill the measuring cup and reserve the rest for later.

Wash the cabbage thoroughly under cold running water and torn with hands. Set aside.

Now, combine potato, artichoke, cucumber, and cabbage in a juicer and process until juiced. Transfer to a serving glass and refrigerate for 10 minutes before serving.

Enjoy!

Nutrition information per serving: Kcal: 150, Protein: 7.7g, Carbs: 47.3g, Fats: 0.4g

18.   Apple Ginger Juice

Ingredients:

1 small Granny Smith's apple, cored

1 small ginger knob, peeled and sliced

1 small pear, cored and chopped

1 small banana, peeled and chunked

1 cup of fresh spinach, chopped

Preparation:

Wash the apple and cut in half. Remove the core and cut into bite-sized pieces. Set aside.

Peel the ginger knob and chop into small pieces. Set aside.

Wash the pear and remove the core. Cut into small pieces and set aside.

Peel the banana and cut into small chunks. Set aside.

Wash the spinach thoroughly under cold running water. Slightly drain and chop into small pieces. Set aside.

Now, combine apple, ginger, pear, banana, and spinach in a juicer and process until juiced. Transfer to a serving glass and refrigerate for 10 minutes before serving.

Enjoy!

Nutrition information per serving: Kcal: 247, Protein: 1.7g, Carbs: 73.9g, Fats: 1.7g

19.   Artichoke Broccoli Juice

Ingredients:

1 medium-sized artichoke, chopped

1 cup of fresh broccoli, chopped

1 cup of Swiss chard, chopped

1 cup of cucumber, sliced

1 oz. of water

Preparation:

Trim off the outer leaves of the artichoke using a sharp paring knife. Wash it and cut into bite-sized pieces. Set aside.

Wash the broccoli and cut into small pieces. Fill the measuring cup and reserve the rest for later. Set aside.

Rinse the Swiss chard under cold running water. Slightly drain and chop into small pieces. Fill the measuring cup and reserve the rest in the refrigerator.

Wash the cucumber and cut into thin slices. Fill the measuring cup and reserve the rest in the refrigerator. Set aside.

Now, combine artichoke, broccoli, Swiss chard, and cucumber in a juicer and process until juiced. Transfer to a serving glass and stir in the water.

Refrigerate for 10 minutes before serving.

Nutrition information per serving: Kcal: 65, Protein: 7.7g, Carbs: 22.7g, Fats: 0.6g

20.   Spinach-Asparagus Juice

Ingredients:

1 cup of fresh spinach, chopped

1 medium-sized wedge of honeydew melon

1 cup of fresh wild asparagus, trimmed and chopped

¼ tsp of ginger, ground

Preparation:

Place the spinach in a colander and wash thoroughly under cold running water. Slightly drain and chop into small pieces. Fill the measuring cup and set aside. Reserve the rest in the refrigerator.

Cut the melon lengthwise in half. Scoop out the seeds and cut one medium-sized wedge. Peel it and cut into bite-sized pieces. Set aside.

Wash the asparagus and trim off the woody ends. Cut into bite-sized pieces and set aside.

Now, combine spinach, melon, and asparagus in a juicer and process until juiced. Transfer to a serving glass and stir in the ginger. Add some ice and serve immediately.

Nutrition information per serving: Kcal: 85, Protein: 9.6g, Carbs: 24.2g, Fats: 1.2g

21. Celery Leek Juice

Ingredients:

2 cups of celery, chopped

1 whole leek, chopped

1 cup of cucumber, sliced

1 cup of fresh basil, chopped

Preparation:

Wash the celery and cut into bite-sized pieces. Fill the measuring cups and reserve the rest for later. Set aside.

Wash the leek and cut into small pieces. Set aside.

Wash the cucumber and cut into thin slices. Fill the measuring cup and reserve the rest for later. Set aside.

Wash the basil thoroughly under cold running water and slightly drain. Chop into small pieces and set aside.

Now, combine celery, leek, cucumber, and basil in a juicer and process until juiced. Transfer to a serving glass and refrigerate for 10 minutes.

Enjoy!

Nutrition information per serving: Kcal: 79, Protein: 3.8g, Carbs: 21.2g, Fats: 0.8g

22.   Coconut Mango Juice

Ingredients:

1 cup of mango, chunked

1 large carrot, sliced

1 small Granny Smith's apple, cored and chopped

1 oz. of coconut water

Preparation:

Peel the mango and cut into chunks. Fill the measuring cup and reserve the rest for later.

Wash and peel the carrot. Cut into bite-sized pieces and set aside.

Wash the apple and cut in half. Remove the core and cut into bite-sized pieces. Set aside.

Now, combine mango, carrot, and apple in a juicer and process until juiced. Transfer to a serving glass and stir in the coconut water. Add some crushed ice and serve immediately.

Enjoy!

Nutrition information per serving: Kcal: 179, Protein: 2.6g, Carbs: 51.2g, Fats: 1.1g

23.   Squash Carrot Juice

Ingredients:

1 cup of butternut squash, cubed

4 baby carrots, sliced

1 cup of green cabbage, chopped

1 cup of cucumber, sliced

¼ tsp of turmeric, ground

Preparation:

Cut the butternut squash lengthwise in half. Scoop out the seeds and cut one large wedge. Peel and chop into small cubes. Wrap the rest of the squash in a plastic foil and place it in the refrigerator.

Wash and peel the carrots. Cut into thin slices and set aside.

Wash the cabbage thoroughly under cold running water. Chop into small pieces and fill the measuring cup. Reserve the rest for later.

Wash the cucumber and cut into thin slices. Fill the measuring cup and reserve the rest for later.

Now, combine squash, carrots, cabbage, and cucumber in a juicer and process until juiced. Transfer to a serving glass and stir in the turmeric.

Refrigerate for 15 minutes before serving.

Nutrition information per serving: Kcal: 108, Protein: 4.1g, Carbs: 35g, Fats: 0.6g

24. Grape Pear Juice

Ingredients:

1 cup of green grapes

1 medium-sized pear, chopped

1 small zucchini, cut into bite-sized cubes

¼ tsp of cinnamon, ground

3 tbsp. of coconut water

Preparation:

Wash the grapes and fill the measuring cup. Set aside.

Wash the pear and cut in half. Remove the core and cut into small pieces. Set aside.

Peel the zucchini and cut into bite-sized cubes. Set aside.

Now, combine grapes, pear, and zucchini in a juicer and process until juiced. Transfer to a serving glass and stir in the cinnamon and coconut water.

Add some crushed ice and serve immediately.

Enjoy!

Nutrition information per serving: Kcal: 153, Protein: 2.6 g, Carbs: 46.6g, Fats: 0.9g

25.   Celery Banana Juice

Ingredients:

1 medium-sized banana, peeled and chunked

1 cup of celery, chopped

1 cup of watermelon, diced

1 oz. of water

Preparation:

Peel the banana and cut into small chunks. Set aside.

Wash the celery and cut into bite-sized pieces. Fill the measuring cup and reserve the rest for later.

Cut the watermelon in half. For one cup, you'll need one large wedge. Peel and dice into small pieces. Remove the pits and fill the measuring cup. Wrap the rest of the melon in a plastic foil and refrigerate for later.

Now, combine banana, celery, and watermelon in a juicer and process until juiced. Transfer to a serving glass and stir in the water.

Add some ice and serve immediately.

Enjoy!

Nutrition information per serving: Kcal: 147, Protein: 2.9g, Carbs: 41.4g, Fats: 0.8g

26. Cabbage Lettuce Juice

Ingredients:

1 cup of green cabbage, chopped

1 cup of Romaine lettuce, chopped

1 cup of broccoli, chopped

1 cup of cucumber, sliced

¼ tsp of salt

Preparation:

Combine cabbage and lettuce in a large colander. Wash thoroughly under cold running water and slightly drain. Chop into small pieces and set aside.

Wash the broccoli and trim off the white part. Cut into bite-sized pieces and fill the measuring cup. Set aside.

Wash the cucumber and cut into thin slices. Fill the measuring cup and reserve the rest in the refrigerator.

Now, combine cabbage, lettuce, broccoli, and cucumber in a juicer and process until well juiced. Transfer to a serving glass and stir in the salt.

Add some ice and serve immediately.

Nutrition information per serving: Kcal: 58, Protein: 5.7g, Carbs: 19.8g, Fats: 0.7g

27. Peach Cantaloupe Juice

Ingredients:

3 medium-sized peaches, pitted and chopped

1 small wedge of cantaloupe

1 cup of pineapple, chunked

¼ tsp of cinnamon, ground

Preparation:

Wash the peaches and cut in half. Remove the pits and cut into bite-sized pieces. Set aside.

Cut the cantaloupe in half and scoop out the seeds. Cut and peel two medium wedges. Fill the measuring cup and reserve the rest for later.

Cut the top of the pineapple and peel it using a sharp paring knife. Peel it all and cut into small pieces. Fill the measuring cup and set aside.

Now, combine peaches, cantaloupe, and pineapple in a juicer and process until juiced. Transfer to a serving glass and stir in the cinnamon.

Refrigerate for 10 minutes before serving.

Nutrition information per serving: Kcal: 237, Protein: 5.4g, Carbs: 69.1g, Fats: 5.4g

28. Guava Carrot Juice

Ingredients:

1 whole guava, chopped

1 medium-sized carrot, sliced

1 cup of cucumber, sliced

1 medium-sized apple, cored and chopped

2 tbsp. of coconut water

Preparation:

Wash the guava and cut into bite-sized pieces. Set aside.

Wash and peel the carrot. Cut into thin slices and set aside.

Wash the cucumber and cut into thin slices. Fill the measuring cup and reserve the rest for later.

Wash the apple and cut in half. Remove the core and cut into bite-sized pieces. Set aside.

Now, combine guava, carrot, cucumber, and apple in a juicer and process until juiced. Transfer to a serving glass and stir in the coconut water.

Add some ice and serve immediately.

Nutrition information per serving: Kcal: 128, Protein: 3.1g, Carbs: 38.3g, Fats: 1.1g

29.   Bean Turnip Juice

Ingredients:

1 cup of green beans, chopped

2 cups of turnip greens, chopped

1 small Granny Smith's apple, chopped

1 cup of cucumber, sliced

1 small ginger knob, peeled and chopped

Preparation:

Wash the beans and place them in a deep pot. Add 2 cups of water and bring it to a boil. Remove from the heat and drain well. Set aside to cool completely and the chop.

Wash the turnip greens thoroughly under cold running water. Chop into small pieces and set aside.

Wash the apple and cut in half. Remove the core and cut into bite-sized pieces. Set aside.

Wash the cucumber and cut into thin slices. Fill the measuring cup and reserve the rest in the refrigerator. Set aside.

Peel the ginger and cut into small pieces. Set aside.

Now, combine beans, turnip greens, apple, cucumber, and ginger in a juicer and process until juiced. Transfer to a serving glass and add few ice cubes.

Serve immediately.

Nutrition information per serving: Kcal: 122, Protein: 3.7g, Carbs: 34.2g, Fats: 0.8g

30.   Spinach Aloe Juice

Ingredients:

1 cup of fresh spinach, chopped

1 cup of fresh kale, chopped

1 cup of cucumber, sliced

1 cup of fennel, chopped

1 tbsp. of aloe vera juice

Preparation:

Combine spinach and kale in a large colander. Wash thoroughly under cold running water and slightly drain. Chop into small pieces and set aside.

Wash the cucumber and cut into thin slices. Fill the measuring cup and reserve the rest for later. Set aside.

Wash the fennel and trim off the green ends. Using a sharp paring knife, remove the outer layer. Cut into small pieces and set aside.

Now, combine spinach, kale, cucumber, and fennel in a juicer and process until juiced. Transfer to a serving glass and stir in the aloe juice.

Refrigerate for 10 minutes before serving.

Nutrition information per serving: Kcal: 74, Protein: 10.3g, Carbs: 34.2g, Fats: 0.8g

31.　Banana Mint Juice

Ingredients:

2 large bananas, peeled and chunked

1 cup of fresh mint, chopped

1 small apple, cored

2 large strawberries, chopped

2 oz. of water

Preparation:

Peel the bananas and cut into small chunks. Set aside.

Wash the mint and roughly chop it. Fill the measuring cup and set aside.

Wash the apple and cut in half. Remove the core and cut into bite-sized pieces. Set aside.

Wash the strawberries and remove the stem. Cut into bite-sized pieces and set aside.

Now, combine bananas, mint, apple, and strawberries in a juicer and process until juiced. Transfer to a serving glass and stir in the water.

Add some ice and serve immediately.

Nutrition information per serving: Kcal: 294, Protein: 4.5g, Carbs: 86.1g, Fats: 1.4g

32.   Chard Pineapple Juice

Ingredients:

2 cups of Swiss chard, chopped

1 cup of pineapple, chunked

1 cup of watermelon, diced

¼ tsp of ginger, ground

Preparation:

Wash the Swiss chard thoroughly under cold running water. Slightly drain and chop into small pieces. Set aside.

Cut the top of the pineapple and peel it using a sharp paring knife. Peel it all and cut into small pieces. Fill the measuring cup and set aside.

Cut the top of the watermelon. Cut lengthwise in half and then cut one large wedge. Peel it and cut into small cubes. Remove the seeds and fill the measuring cup. Wrap the rest in a plastic foil and refrigerate for later.

Now, combine Swiss chard, pineapple, and watermelon in a juicer and process until juiced. Transfer to a serving glass and stir in the ginger.

Add some ice and serve immediately.

Nutrition information per serving: Kcal: 127, Protein: 3.1g, Carbs: 35.8g, Fats: 0.6g

33.   Sprout Cauliflower Juice

Ingredients:

2 cups of Brussels sprouts, halved

1 cup of cauliflower, chopped

1 cup of cucumber, sliced

1 cup of mustard greens, torn

1 oz of water

Preparation:

Wash the Brussels sprouts and trim off the wilted leaves. Cut each sprout in half and fill the measuring cup. Reserve the rest for later.

Trim off the outer leaves of the outer leaves of a cauliflower. Cut into bite-sized pieces and fill the measuring cup. Reserve the rest for later.

Wash the cucumber and cut into thin slices. Fill the measuring cup and reserve the rest in the refrigerator.

Wash the mustard greens thoroughly under cold running water. Slightly drain and chop into small pieces. Set aside.

Now, combine Brussels sprouts, cauliflower, cucumber, and mustard greens in a juicer and process until juiced. Transfer to a serving glass and stir in the water.

Enjoy!

Nutrition information per serving: Kcal: 91, Protein: 10.3g, Carbs: 27.5g, Fats: 1.1g

34.   Strawberry Watermelon Juice

Ingredients:

8 large strawberries, chopped

1 cup of watermelon, diced

1 cup of fresh mint, torn

1 small Granny Smith's apple, core and chopped

¼ tsp of cinnamon, ground

Preparation:

Wash the strawberries and remove the stems. Cut into bite-sized pieces and set aside.

Cut the top of the watermelon. Cut lengthwise in half and then cut one large wedge. Peel the wedge and cut into small cubes. Remove the seeds and fill the measuring cup. Wrap the rest in a plastic foil and refrigerate.

Wash the mint thoroughly and slightly drain. Torn with hands and set aside.

Wash the apple and cut in half. Remove the core and cut into bite-sized pieces. Set aside.

Now, combine strawberries, watermelon, mint, and apple in a juicer and process until juiced. Transfer to a serving glass and stir in the cinnamon.

Add some crushed ice and serve immediately.

Nutrition information per serving: Kcal: 154, Protein: 3.5g, Carbs: 45.8g, Fats: 1.1g

35. Apricot Apple Juice

Ingredients:

3 whole apricots, chopped

1 small apple, chopped

1 medium-sized banana, sliced

1 medium-sized celery stalk, chopped

Preparation:

Wash the apricots and cut in half. Remove the pits and cut into bite-sized pieces. Set aside.

Wash the apple and cut in half. Remove the core and cut into bite-sized pieces. Set aside.

Peel the banana and cut into small chunks. Set aside.

Wash the celery stalk and cut into bite-sized pieces. Set aside.

Now, combine apricots, apple, banana, and celery in a juicer and process until juiced. Transfer to a serving glass and add some ice.

Serve immediately.

Nutrition information per serving: Kcal: 154, Protein: 3.5g, Carbs: 45.8g, Fats: 1.1g

36.   Zucchini Parsnip Juice

Ingredients:

1 small zucchini, chopped

1 cup of parsnip, sliced

1 cup of watercress, chopped

1 cup of cucumber, sliced

Preparation:

Peel the zucchini and cut into thin slices. Set aside.

Wash the parsnip and trim off the green parts. Slightly peel and cut into slices. Set side.

Wash the watercress thoroughly under cold running water. Drain and chop into small pieces. Set aside.

Wash the cucumber and cut into thin slices. Fill the measuring cup and reserve the rest for later. Set aside.

Now, combine zucchini, parsnip, watercress, and cucumber in a juicer and process until juiced. Transfer to a serving glass and stir in the water.

Add some ice and serve immediately.

Nutrition information per serving: Kcal: 99, Protein: 4.2g, Carbs: 29.9g, Fats: 0.9g

37.   Radish Leek Juice

Ingredients:

5 large radishes, chopped

2 whole leeks, chopped

2 cups of cucumber, sliced

2 cups of red leaf lettuce, shredded

1 cup of asparagus, trimmed

Preparation:

Wash the radishes and trim off the green parts. Slightly peel and cut into thin slices. Set aside.

Wash the leeks and cut into bite-sized pieces. Set aside.

Wash the cucumber and cut into thin slices. Fill the measuring cups and reserve the rest in the refrigerator.

Wash the lettuce thoroughly under cold running water. Shred it and fill the measuring cups. Reserve the rest for later.

Wash the asparagus and trim off the woody ends. Cut into bite-sized pieces and set aside.

Now, combine radishes, leeks, cucumber, lettuce, and asparagus in a juicer and process until juiced. Transfer to a serving glass and add some crushed ice before serving.

Enjoy!

Nutrition information per serving: Kcal: 137, Protein: 7.3g, Carbs: 37g, Fats: 1g

38. Honeydew Melon Avocado Juice

Ingredients:

1 large wedge of honeydew melon, chopped

1 cup of avocado, cubed

1 cup of mango, chopped

1 small ginger knob, sliced

1 oz of water

Preparation:

Cut the melon in half. Cut one large wedge and peel the peel it. Cut into small pieces and set aside. Wrap the rest of the melon in a plastic foil and refrigerate for later.

Peel the avocado and cut lengthwise in half. Remove the pit and cut into small cubes. Fill the measuring cup and reserve the rest in the refrigerator.

Peel the mango and chop into bite-sized pieces. Fill the measuring cup and reserve the rest in the refrigerator.

Peel the ginger knob and cut it in small pieces. Set aside.

Now, combine melon, avocado, mango, and ginger in a juicer and process until well juiced. Transfer to a serving glass and stir in the water.

Add some ice and serve immediately.

Enjoy!

Nutrition information per serving: Kcal: 347, Protein: 5.3g, Carbs: 53.1g, Fats: 22.8g

39.   Crookneck Squash Juice

Ingredients:

1 cup of crookneck squash, cubed

1 cup of pumpkin, chopped

1 cup of cucumber, sliced

¼ tsp of turmeric, ground

¼ tsp of salt

2 tbsp. of water

Preparation:

Cut the squash lengthwise in half. Using a teaspoon, scoop out the seeds and clean it inside. Peel and cut into small cubes. Fill the measuring cup and wrap the rest in a plastic foil and refrigerate.

Peel the pumpkin and cut lengthwise in half. Scoop out the seeds and cut into small cubes. Fill the measuring cup and reserve the rest in the refrigerator.

Wash the cucumber and cut into thin slices. Fill the measuring cup and reserve the rest in the refrigerator.

Now, combine squash, pumpkin, and cucumber in a juicer and process until juiced. Transfer to a serving glass and stir in the turmeric, salt, and water.

Refrigerate for 10 minutes before serving.

Nutrition information per serving: Kcal: 73, Protein: 4.1g, Carbs: 19.3g, Fats: 0.9g

40.   Basil Avocado Juice

Ingredients:

1 cup of fresh basil, chopped

1 cup of avocado, cubed

1 small Granny Smith's apple, cored

1 small peach, chopped

1 oz. of water

Preparation:

Wash the basil thoroughly under cold running water. Slightly drain and chop into small pieces. Set aside.

Peel the avocado and cut in half. Remove the pit and cut into small cubes. Fill the measuring cup and reserve the rest for later.

Wash the apple and cut lengthwise in half. Remove the core and cut into bite-sized pieces. Set aside.

Wash the peach and cut in half. Remove the pit and chop into small pieces. Set aside.

Now, combine basil, avocado, apple, and peach in a juicer and process until well juiced. Transfer to a serving glass and stir in the water.

Add some ice and serve immediately.

Enjoy!

Nutrition information per serving: Kcal: 315, Protein: 5.6g, Carbs: 45.4g, Fats: 22.7g

41.   Carrot Pineapple Juice

Ingredients:

1 large carrot, sliced

1 cup of pineapple, chunked

1 cup of blackberries

1 oz. of water

Preparation:

Wash and peel the carrot. Cut into bite-sized pieces and set aside.

Using a sharp paring knife, cut the top of a pineapple and the peel it completely. Cut into small chunks and fill the measuring cup. Reserve the rest for later. Set aside.

Wash the blackberries using a colander. Slightly drain and set aside.

Now, combine carrot, pineapple, and blackberries in a juicer and process until juiced. Transfer to a serving glass and stir in the water.

Add some ice and serve immediately.

Nutrition information per serving: Kcal: 127, Protein: 3.6g, Carbs: 42.4g, Fats: 1.1g

42.   Potato Ginger Juice

Ingredients:

1 cup of sweet potatoes, chunked

1 ginger knob, sliced

1 large carrot, sliced

1 cup of cucumber, sliced

2 oz. of water

Preparation:

Peel the potato and cut into small chunks. Fill the measuring cup and reserve the rest for later. Set aside.

Peel the ginger knob and cut into thin slices. Set aside.

Wash and peel the carrot. Cut into thin slices and set aside.

Wash the cucumber and cut into thin slices. Fill the measuring cup and reserve the rest for later.

Now, combine potato, ginger, carrot, and cucumber in a juicer and process until juiced transfer to a serving glass and stir in the water.

Nutrition information per serving: Kcal: 132, Protein: 3.2g, Carbs: 36.6g, Fats: 0.4g

43.   Pear Raspberry Juice

Ingredients:

2 medium-sized pears, chopped

1 cup of cucumber, sliced

1 medium-sized banana, sliced

1 cup of raspberries

Preparation:

Wash the pear and cut in half. Remove the core and cut into bite-sized pieces. Set aside.

Wash the cucumber and cut into thin slices. Fill the measuring cup and reserve the rest for later.

Peel the banana and cut into small chunks. Set aside.

Wash the raspberries using a colander. Slightly drain and set aside.

Now, combine pear, cucumber, banana, and raspberries in a juicer and process until juiced. Transfer to a serving glass and add some crushed ice.

Nutrition information per serving: Kcal: 290, Protein: 4.4g, Carbs: 97.7g, Fats: 1.8g

44.   Papaya Mint Juice

Ingredients:

1 large papaya, chopped

1 cup of fresh mint, chopped

1 small Granny Smith's apple, cored

1 tbsp. of coconut water

Preparation:

Peel the papaya and cut lengthwise in half. Scoop out the seeds and chop into small pieces. Set aside.

Wash the mint thoroughly under cold running water. Chop into small pieces and set aside.

Wash the apple and cut in half. Remove the core and cut into bite-sized pieces. Set aside.

Now, combine papaya, mint, and apple in a juicer and process until juiced. Transfer to a serving glass and stir in the coconut water.

Refrigerate for 10 minutes before serving.

Nutrition information per serving: Kcal: 290, Protein: 4.4g, Carbs: 97.7g, Fats: 1.8g

45.   Chamomile Juice

Ingredients:

1 tsp of chamomile tea

2 large carrots, sliced

1 cup of watermelon, diced

1 cup of cucumber, sliced

2 tbsp. of hot water

¼ tsp of ginger, ground

Preparation:

Combine chamomile and hot water in a small cup or a bowl. Soak for 5 minutes. Set aside.

Wash and peel the carrots. Cut into thin slices and set aside.

Cut the top of the watermelon. Cut lengthwise in half and then cut one large wedge. Peel it and dice into small pieces. Remove the seeds and fill the measuring cup. Wrap the rest in a plastic foil and refrigerate for later.

Wash the cucumber and cut into thin slices. Fill the measuring cup and reserve the rest for later. Set aside.

Now, combine chamomile mixture, carrots, watermelon, and cucumber in a juicer and process until juiced.

Transfer to a serving glass and stir in the ginger. Refrigerate for 10 minutes before serving.

Enjoy!

Nutrition information per serving: Kcal: 96, Protein: 2.6g, Carbs: 27.2g, Fats: 0.6g

46. Apple Aloe Juice

Ingredients:

1 small Granny Smith's apple, cored

1 tbsp. of aloe juice

1 cup of cucumber, sliced

1 medium-sized banana, sliced

1 large celery stalk, chopped

Preparation:

Wash the apple and cut in half. Remove the core and cut into bite-sized pieces. Set aside.

Wash the cucumber and cut into thin slices. Fill the measuring cup and reserve the rest for later. Set aside.

Peel the banana and cut into chunks. Set aside.

Wash the celery stalk and chop into bite-sized pieces. Set aside.

Now, combine apple, cucumber, banana, and celery in a juicer. Process until juiced.

Transfer to a serving glass and stir in the aloe juice.

Add some crushed ice and serve immediately.

Nutrition information per serving: Kcal: 174, Protein: 2.7g, Carbs: 50.3g, Fats: 0.8g

## 47.	Avocado Zucchini Juice

Ingredients:

1 cup of avocado, cubed

1 medium-sized zucchini

1 whole leek, chopped

2 medium-sized asparagus spears

3 tbsp. of water

Preparation:

Peel the avocado and cut lengthwise in half. Remove the core and cut into small cubes. Fill the measuring cup and reserve the rest in the refrigerator.

Peel the zucchini and cut into bite-sized pieces. Set aside.

Wash the leek and cut into small pieces. Set aside.

Now, combine avocado, zucchini, leek, and asparagus in a juicer and process until juiced. Transfer to a serving glass and stir in the water.

Refrigerate for 10 minutes before serving.

Nutrition information per serving: Kcal: 277, Protein: 22.9g, Carbs: 32.7g, Fats: 22.9g

48.   Pineapple Mint Juice

Ingredients:

1 cup of pineapple, chunked

1 cup of fresh mint, torn

1 cup of watercress, chopped

1 cup of Romaine lettuce, torn

¼ tsp of ginger, ground

Preparation:

Cut the top of the pineapple and peel it using a sharp paring knife. Peel it and cut into small pieces. Set aside.

Combine watercress, mint, and lettuce in a large colander. Wash thoroughly under cold running water and torn into small pieces. Set aside.

Now, combine pineapple, mint, watercress, and lettuce in a juicer. Process until juiced.

Transfer to a serving glass and add some ice before serving.

Nutrition information per serving: Kcal: 90, Protein: 3.2g, Carbs: 27.3g, Fats: 0.6g

49.   Melon Ginger Juice

Ingredients:

1 cup of watermelon, diced

1 medium-sized wedge of honeydew melon

1 small ginger knob, peeled and chopped

1 medium-sized carrot, sliced

1 small banana, chunked

Preparation:

Cut the top of the watermelon. Cut lengthwise in half and then cut one large wedge. Peel it and cut into small cubes. Remove the seeds and fill the measuring cup. Wrap the rest in a plastic foil and refrigerate for later.

Cut the melon in half. Cut one large wedge and peel the peel it. Cut into small pieces and set aside. Wrap the rest of the melon in a plastic foil and refrigerate for some other juice.

Peel the ginger and cut into small pieces. Set aside.

Wash and peel the carrot. Cut into thin slices and set aside.

Peel the banana and cut into chunks. Set aside.

Now, combine watermelon, honeydew melon, ginger, carrot, and banana in a juicer. Process until juiced.

Transfer to a serving glass and add some crushed ice before serving.

Nutrition information per serving: Kcal: 188, Protein: 3.4g, Carbs: 52.8g, Fats: 0.9g

50.   Pear Cucumber Juice

Ingredients:

1 medium-sized pear, cored

1 cup of cucumber, sliced

1 cup of kale, torn

1 small green apple, cored

Preparation:

Wash the pear and cut lengthwise in half. Remove the core and cut into bite-sized pieces.

Wash the cucumber and cut into thin slices. Fill the measuring cup and reserve the rest for later. Set aside.

Wash the kale thoroughly under cold running water and slightly drain. Torn with hands and set aside.

Wash the apple and remove the core. Cut into small pieces and set aside.

Now, combine pear, cucumber, kale, and apple in a juicer and process until juiced. Transfer to a serving glass and add some ice before serving.

Nutrition information per serving: Kcal: 177, Protein: 4.4g, Carbs: 54.5g, Fats: 1.2g

ADDITIONAL TITLES FROM THIS AUTHOR

70 Effective Meal Recipes to Prevent and Solve Being Overweight: Burn Fat Fast by Using Proper Dieting and Smart Nutrition

By Joe Correa CSN

48 Acne Solving Meal Recipes: The Fast and Natural Path to Fixing Your Acne Problems in Less Than 10 Days!

By Joe Correa CSN

41 Alzheimer's Preventing Meal Recipes: Reduce or Eliminate Your Alzheimer's Condition in 30 Days or Less!

By Joe Correa CSN

70 Effective Breast Cancer Meal Recipes: Prevent and Fight Breast Cancer with Smart Nutrition and Powerful Foods

By Joe Correa CSN